MAN IN THE MIRROR:
CHALLENGE YOURSELF EVERY DAY TO BECOME
THE ULTIMATE VERSION OF THE MAN INSIDE

BY

JESSE EWELL

MAN IN THE MIRROR

Ordering Information: Quantity sales. Special discounts are available on quantity purchases by corporations, associations, and others. Orders by U.S. trade bookstores and wholesalers. Please contact Jesse Ewell, www.habitbasedlifestyle.com, jesse@habitbasedlifestyle.com.

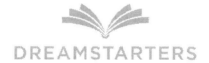

Edited and Marketed By DreamStarters University
www.DreamStartersUniversity.com

Foreword by Sam Falsafi

It has been almost four years since I first saw Jesse Ewell in the ring, boxing, full of blood, one fight after another one, never stopping. Jesse refused to stop because he was fighting for a purpose. He was fighting for his family and he was fighting for his wife. For the first time ever, Jesse found the clarity of *why* he was actually winning in life and why he wanted to win.

For most of his life, Jesse has been a very competitive guy, and inside that experience, winning was always his target. No matter what, Jesse had to win. For his first time ever, four years ago, inside of a boxing ring, with his bloody nose, and his opponent on the floor, Jesse raised his head and he said, "I know why I must win now. I'm winning for my wife, for my kids, and for myself." And that declaration is true to this day, four years later.

Four years after that declaration, Jesse Ewell fights every single day for himself first, and then for his wife and his kids. He's created habits and routines that allow him to win at the game of life. Through living the warrior's way, he's created a life of growth, expansion, and prosperity, by pushing himself every day to become a better version of himself. Jesse Ewell is a man that does not accept the image of what he saw in the mirror yesterday. Every day he looks at himself in the mirror, and every day he wants to win.

And so this book is going to give you the path and the guidance towards the system of the matrix, the ideology, the psychology, the heart, the energy, the mind, and the body. More importantly, this book will show you the soul of a man. A man who knows he wants to win for his wife, for his kids, for his family, but most of all, for himself.

For the first time ever, you're going to read a book that will give you permission to make yourself a priority. To put yourself *first* when you look in the mirror, before you start seeing the images of other people. The reflections of others do not mean anything if you cannot see yourself as the man in the mirror.

The modern man today can't look always look at himself in the mirror. The modern man has become a slave to other people's opinions. The modern man has become a good man rather than being good at being a man. Being a good man is a nice slave; he makes a good slave.

Being good at being a man is a whole different chapter and agenda. That's what you're going to discover in this book. In this book, each chapter is going to lead and unlock the path to becoming good at being a man, and not simply tolerating being good.

So as you read these chapters, and as you get to know the story of Jesse Ewell, know that he's found the light in the night and you too, my friend, can turn on the light in the night if you simply give yourself permission to follow the path of the enlightened.

It is my honor and my duty as a brother and a friend, as family, to continue to see Jesse Ewell rise and support him in the verse. He's a friend, he's a brother, he's a leader. He is Jesse Ewell, a fucking winner.

When you enter this book, I advise that you grasp from the heart. As you read, I encourage you to feel this book and connect with the heart of Jesse Ewell. Know where his heart is, because when you understand this concept, you begin seeking something that is seeking you.

Inside that experience, you find the guidance and the enlightenment that you have been looking for. This guidance does not come through the words of Jesse Ewell, but Jesse Ewell simply acts as an instrument. He will be the environment for you to give yourself an opportunity to finally listen to the voice inside of you. What's inside you paints an image of possibility in your life, and that will guide you through the chapters and words in this book. You'll gain knowledge of possibility in your life and the ultimate patterns and habits that need to let go of.

This new routine that needs to be created for you, will enable you to rise to the targets you envision. Allow yourself to navigate through these chapters and connect not to the words of Jesse Ewell, not to the structure of the chapters, not in how it's written, but to the simplicity of the message that resonates in your heart.

In this place, in this book, there is a gift for you. The question remains: what will you do in order to go and get this gift? Will you decide to read a few pages and come back for more later? Will you buy the book and put it on the shelf? Or will you truly give yourself the permission to go all in and find what the gift may be inside of the book?

When you do, it is then that you realize that there is a divine gift waiting for you. I'm excited for you as you read the chapters of this book, because the man that I know, Jesse Ewell, the man that I believe can guide you as a shepherd to this gift, is already giving away the gift that he's received to so many other men. I have been the witness of that, so go ahead my friend, allow these words to warm your heart.

Acknowledgement

No matter how successful we are in life and business, no one person is self-made. Over my 40 years I've had so many people help me, I want to personally acknowledge you.

Before anyone else, I would like to thank my wife, Katie, who has been the most supportive person in my life throughout the last 14 years. You have played every role a person can play: spouse, friend, business partner, critic, supporter, fan, and more than anything else, you believed in me long before I believed in me. I could not and would not be where I am today without you by my side. We did all of this together as a team.

Second, I'm grateful for my kids, Taylor, Jesse Jr., Julia, and Jocelyn. My kids have taught me so much about myself and bring me joy and happiness. The special moments of coaching football, going on dates, wrestling in the living room, and coming home after a long day at work, have a special place in my heart. Without all of you, I would not have a mission to leave a legacy. This book is as much for you as anyone else.

I'm grateful for my family. It's hard to tell the truth about what happened as a kid and teenager, but it has also liberated me and brought me to understand myself and my parents on a much deeper level. I have to thank my parents for all their years of support, and for always wanting what they believed was best for me. Thank you for your teaching me the definition of hard work, for showing up at all my sporting events, and for the sacrifices you made. I want my mom Brenda, dad Bob, and brother Jake, to know I deeply love them.

I would also like to thank my father- and mother-in-law, Mike and Teri, for supporting and investing into our business long before anyone else believed. You taught me the lesson of what it means to leave a legacy, and how it can impact generations to come.

At various stages of life, people cross your paths and play important roles. I would like to thank two men who have played major roles in my life, Garret J. White, for creating the first program for Masculinity and Married Business Men. Previously, there was no blueprint on how to be a modern man but Wake up Warrior has taught me so much about being a husband, father, leader, and businessman. I'm forever grateful for this program and the personal sacrifice you have made to create it.

I would also like to thank my brother Sam Falsafi. He was the first man to reach out to me from Warrior, and since our first conversation, we have been brothers ever since. Your friendship, brotherhood, and support are truly appreciated.

Next goes out to the many family members, cousins, uncles, aunts, friends, clients, co-workers and people who have impacted me. Through our experiences together, interactions, stories, and your ability to open up and share, I would not be the man I am today without all of you.

To every mentor, teacher, coach, and trainer I've had, you have all inspired me to be the man I am today.

Special thanks go out to Mike Fallat for writing this book and putting my thoughts and stories on paper. It has been a pleasure working with you.

There are always people left off the list, and if you're not on here, consider yourself a friend or family member. This book has to stop somewhere and who knows? Maybe more books will be written in the future where your name will show up. Until then I will leave you with this.....

The Man In The Glass

When you get what you want in your struggle for self

And the world makes you king for a day

Just go to the mirror and look at yourself

And see what that man has to say.

For it isn't your father, or mother, or wife

Whose judgment upon you must pass

The fellow whose verdict counts most in your life

Is the one staring back from the glass.

He's the fellow to please – never mind all the rest

For he's with you, clear to the end

And you've passed your most difficult, dangerous test

If the man in the glass is your friend.

You may fool the whole world down the pathway of years

And get pats on the back as you pass

But your final reward will be heartache and tears

If you've cheated the man in the glass.

Peter Dale Wimbrow Sr.

"As long as we persevere and endure, we can get anything we want."

Mike Tyson

This book is for the man you are, were, and want to become.

Right now, he might be asleep.

He might be buried.

He might be forgotten.

He might be lost.

He might have failed.

He might be hurt.

He might have given up.

He might be "dead."

...But if you're reading this, you still have time to turn it all around.

The following pages will show you there is only one way to be truly proud of the man in the mirror. That is to challenge yourself daily, level-up on all fronts, and never stop searching for the ultimate version of the man inside.

Table of Contents

Chapter 1

Commitment to Consistency

What are you committed to in life? What drives you to focus, to learn, to improve? I am committed to constant growth. No matter how difficult or painful the journey may be, constant growth is what drives me to do what I do. This level of unprecedented, unwavering commitment provides me with purpose and drive every single day.

Commitment to growth has transitioned me from the man I *was*, to the man I *am*, and to the man I will *become*.

My name is Jesse Ewell. I am a husband, a father, an entrepreneur, a personal trainer, a coach, and a Warrior. My life hasn't always gone as expected, but through trials, tribulations and connecting with influential mentors, I have found *myself* and *my soul purpose.*

My goal is to strengthen and empower you to achieve ultimate levels of success and happiness in your life. I challenge myself every day to be the best person I can be and will push you to do the same.

The importance of commitment was impressed upon me early in life. I started boxing at nine years old, and it led to my nearly 30-year commitment of working hard and working out.

The idea to box came from my buddy's dad. This was back when *Rocky* was out -- it was a big deal at the time.

As a child, I lived in Spokane, WA. On two and three nights a week, we would get dropped off about a mile from our boxing club in one of the worst areas of town. We would run through the shitty weather and the bad part of town just to get to our boxing club. I did this for about six or seven years.

We were around guys who were in Olympic trials, on the U.S. Junior Olympic team, so seeing other guys that were successful in our boxing club pushed us even more. As a child, these mentors were incredibly motivating and inspiring.

Boxing was the first time in life that I had a real coach. I'd go into the ring, and he would tactically break down what I was doing, how I was going to strategize, and how I was going to show up in the next round. This skill helped in other sports because I'd break down what I had done in games, and then analyzed exactly what I needed to do to improve.

My coaches pushed me way harder than if I was doing it on my own. What I remember the most from back then, was the immense amount of work we put into this. At only nine years old, I was doing shit that people weren't doing until age 16 or 17.

Training was difficult. The conditioning aspect of it included running, pushups, sit-ups, weights, boxing drills, and nutrition -- you couldn't just eat whatever you wanted. I remember eating steak that my dad made, chewing it up, sucking the juice out, and then having to spit it out. I was that committed.

The boxing club experience shaped the way that I showed up in other sports such as baseball, wrestling, track and field, and football. In high school, I became an all-state football player, which led to my ultimate goal -- playing football in junior college.

This regular boxing commitment also began my introduction to lifting weights, which shaped my development over the next 20 years in the personal training industry. Boxing also taught me about the amount of work you have to put into something. I quickly learned that **what you put into something is exactly what you're going to get out of it**.

I'd say that the biggest life skill that boxing teaches is that when you get hit, *you get back up*. When I got hit it, it only pushed me to hit back harder. Although young, I was big and husky for my age, so I was boxing guys two and three years older than me. Naturally there was this factor of, "Oh shit, I'm fighting these older guys," but it forced me to show up and play at a higher level. Not only was I scared to get in the ring, but I was fighting these older guys who weighed more than me. I didn't back down and got in the ring anyway.

I'll admit, I was always afraid of fighting. Before a boxing match or a football game, I would dry heave and get sick. I was always terrified to fight until the first punch was thrown, and then I got in the zone. I managed to find a calm headspace and was all in after that first punch.

This fear of the unknown and my resulting physical reaction always pushed me to continue to train. Whether I was boxing or playing a different sport, *I was always acting.* Because of my consistency, I was always doing something physically active.

In my family, if I wasn't playing a sport I was working side-by-side with my dad at our house. My parents had 30 acres of land, so there was constantly work that needed to be done on our property.

I would periodically take off time from a sport, but it was usually over the summer, or to play a different sport. And sometimes I did two sports at once. I was always disciplined and took care of my physical health.

Although I was matched against those older than I was, I was never beat in a match. There was one time during the Washington State Winter Games, where I decided to fight after taking about nine months off. Before the fight, my opponent was talking shit to me before getting into the ring.

"I'm going to kick your ass," he said. I decided to keep to myself, didn't say anything, and when we got to it, I knocked him out through the ring ropes where they broke in the first round. I won Outstanding Boxer of that tournament. Although I was intimidated because he was talking shit and I had taken time off, I was grateful for my training beforehand and active lifestyle, that helped me pull out a win.

Boxing is truly an art and I love it. Some of my favorite boxers are Mike Tyson, Evander Holyfield, Julio César Chávez, Roberto Durán, and Thomas Hearns. Each fighter has his own individual style. Some are power punchers, some are defensive fighters, and others are more offensive. My favorites are the guys like me who stand in the middle of the ring and slug it out. It's a mentality that, "I will give you everything I've got, and you'll give me everything you've got."

That's how I would identify myself -- as someone who is willing to go toe-to-toe with anyone else.

I don't box anymore but maintain my active lifestyle. I currently do Krav Maga, an Israeli military self-defense program that basically takes every martial art, boxing, kickboxing, knife and gun defense, and puts it in a blender.

I've applied what I learned from boxing for the last 28 years of my life, and I feel this consistency has brought me to where I am today. The reason that I got into excellent shape was not because of a specific workout, it was because of *consistency*. I've worked out for 28 years straight because of my consistency and commitment to a daily habit.

I take these lessons and leverage them in all areas of my life. In fact, the art of consistency inside my marriage has completely changed and improved my relationship with my wife.

Is there something positive in your life that is the direct result of consistency or commitment? I want you to look at the things you need to do to challenge yourself. Look at your physical side and your psyche, and challenge yourself in an area to grow and go to the next level. My book will show you how.

By the time you finish this, I want you to feel committed to your personal growth, to discovering the ultimate version of you, and to live your best possible life. Today is your day to embark on an exciting new mission.

CHALLENGE YOURSELF

Everybody is consistent at something. Even if it's a harmful or wasteful habit, we're still consistent at doing these things on a daily basis. Take five minutes to write down a list of things that you have committed to being consistent to. Once written down, take a look at what serves you and what doesn't. What are you doing on a daily basis that is working for you, and what are you doing on a daily basis that is working against you? Just by becoming aware, you begin to see the things you can change.

_____
_____
_____
_____
_____
_____
_____
_____
_____
_____
_____
_____
_____

"The difference between me and a lot of other people is the fact that I just don't stop. It's not that I'm exceptionally talented at what I do; I've just become committed to not stopping."

Garrett J. White

Chapter 2

Daily Habits

Let's talk wake-up calls -- those moments in your life where suddenly everything shifts into view and your entire outlook changes. Have you had one or more of these in your life? ***These massive moments of clarity rely on recognition and action.*** You have to do something with this information and new perspective, otherwise you're doomed to stay stagnant in life.

Getting punched in the face is exactly what led me to change my life.

As Mike Tyson said, "Everybody has a plan until they get punched in the mouth." I found myself in exactly that position. I thought I was successfully handling my life and taking care of my responsibilities, but it turns out that I was neglecting much. The life I was leading was completely two-dimensional.

I'm going to tell you the story about the moment that everything changed for me. And of how that moment saved my life as I know it, all because I chose to take action.

It was 2014, and my marriage was falling apart. We were having so many issues because my wife felt like she wasn't understood or heard. At the time, I was working until 8 p.m. each night, running our personal training facility, and we had two young kids. My wife and I got lost in the chaos and we became completely disconnected.

During this time, I discovered **Wake Up Warrior**, the world's #1 training for married businessmen. I filled out an online application and then made my scheduled follow-up phone call. I remember waiting on hold from 7 p.m. to 11 p.m. waiting to talk to its founder, Garrett J. White. I thought that this lengthy hold time was a test, so I hung in there as long as I could before I finally hung up. I told myself that this must have not been the right time in my life and accepted it for what I thought it was.

A couple months went by and my marriage only got worse. I'll never forget the day that I received a call from my wife, because she was crying so hard that I could barely understand her. She asked me to meet her at her counselor's office.

All I could remember was how *pissed* I was that I had to be off work to deal with this. I walked into the office, sat down, and the counselor looked at me and said, "Do you have any idea what's going on?" What I hadn't realized was that my wife was dying on the inside and could not talk to me, fearing I would leave her. In that moment I realized I had to do something. I thought, "I just want to find a way to change all of this."

Two weeks later, one of the guys from Wake Up Warrior, Sam Falsafi, reached out to me. He noticed that I filled out an application a few months prior but didn't have my phone call. I told him about waiting on hold for four hours, and he apologized explaining that it was an issue with their system. He said, "Anybody who's that committed needs to be on the phone right now with Garrett," and he put me straight through.

I can remember Garrett asking me a very straight question that stopped me in my tracks. He asked, "If you treated your business like you treated your wife, how successful would your business be?" My first thought was that I would barely be paying the bills. So five minutes later, I committed to Warrior Week, which was set for February. I was looking forward to some positive changes in my life.

Not soon after, life threw two major curveballs on the same day. It was the end of December 2015, and I had just fired one of my best friends who happened to be one of my managers of my gym. Shortly after, I received a phone call informing me that my grandma had just died. About an hour later, I got a phone call from Sam at Wake Up Warrior saying, "Hey man, we need you to come to Warrior Week in two weeks. We have a spot for you and you got to come in."

Although the timing didn't seem great, and I knew very little about Warrior Week, I knew that I wanted to be there, so I agreed to attending sooner than I expected.

Along came January and it was time for what would be my first of many experiences with Wake Up Warrior. I went into Warrior Week for the purpose of business, as many people do, and within an hour of being there, I realized that I was going in there for my *marriage*.

One of the first activities was boxing. This took me back in time, but **the moment I got punched in the face, it woke me up again**. I asked myself, "What the fuck have you been doing the last two years with your wife, not paying attention to her and not being connected?"

That punch in the face was just what I needed.

That same day, I learned about Warrior's Core-4 daily habits, which cover Body, Being, Balance, and Business. After getting punched in the face, I woke up and realized I had been living only a 1- or 2-dimensional lifestyle. I was only focusing on Body and Business, but was skipping out on Balance and Being. I thought, "Well shit, I already do fitness and fuel my body, now I can start doing these other habits and round out the rest of my life."

My excuse was that I was building the business and earning money, so I didn't really know what my wife's problem was. Within the first hour of Warrior Week, I realized I was part of the problem in my relationships, and that I hadn't been showing up as a husband. Yes, I was making money, but that was not fulfilling my wife.

Here's a quick breakdown of the daily habits as part of Core-4. **Body** is all about your fitness and how you fuel your body. **Being** covers meditation, prayer, connecting with God and yourself, and journaling your experiences. **Balance** is all about giving daily messages of love, and honoring and appreciating others. **Business** focuses on how to discover, read, and learn something every day, and how to declare something out into social media, teaching someone else.

As an entrepreneur there was no balance. I focused mostly on business and thought I was doing the right thing. Warrior Week helped me realize that I have to focus on more than just one aspect of my life, because the others were suffering.

I realized that there are certain things I can do so that my family knows I love them every day. And there are things I could do to connect to God, and not just on Sundays while taking the other six days off.

I began to consistently go through these Core-4 habits every day, and it really started shaping the next few years for me. As I said, all I was showing up in was barely my Body and Business because that's all I could handle at the time.

After adding new habits, I felt massive growth, a deeper connection with my wife, and I felt like my purpose changed. I came to the conclusion that it wasn't just about making money, it was about being connected to my family, knowing my purpose, being connected to God, having a deeper relationship, and feeling like I was living in balance.

My wife and I went on dates every week, I left her video messages every day, and have continued this for the past four years. Every single day, I'll shoot a video and send it to her saying something like, "Hey this is how I'm feeling about you today and where we're at," *within the framework of honor, love and appreciation*. As I did this and was more present, my wife started to change herself and how *she* showed up. She knew where I was every day and how we were, and this opened up our communication on new levels.

I also started recording videos for my kids, and they started leaving them for me -- it changed our family.

After Warrior Week, I added in mediation and learned how to slow down and create space in my life so that I could be more focused and present. I realized that at home I was thinking about work, and at work I was thinking about home.

Mediation gave me the ability to be present and focus. We call it "being connected to the voice," referring to the one that you hear in your head and listening to it with clarity. Because of meditation, I feel more connected to God and to the voice, and as a result, I make better decisions.

This is what we teach and do with Wake Up Warrior. I break down someone's behaviors and habits so that they are in synch with their outcomes and targets. This is part of the Warrior lifestyle and breaking these habits down to lineup with what you want over the next 90 days or the next year is the key. Our guidance will have you setting new outcomes and targets that will ultimately lead you to the person you want to become in the next year.

A lot of men lose their purpose, they're just working and not necessarily living their purpose. If all you're doing is working for money, after a while it doesn't really fulfill you. We do stuff to make money, but it doesn't align with our purpose. Meshing in with what fulfills us takes us to the highest level, and I want you to experience this for yourself.

I encourage you to visualize where you want to be and who you want to become, as according to the Core-4 values.

I am so grateful that I was open to Wake Up Warrior, that I recognized I needed a change, and that -- yes -- I was punched in the face. All of these changes started with me, but I continued to be open, to learn, and to take the disciplined steps by creating new, healthy, daily habits.

CHALLENGE YOURSELF

Ask yourself who you want to become in the next year over the categories of Body, Being, Balance and Business. Now break these down into who you want to become in the next 90 days. What beliefs and identities must change in order to pull this off? What fear and lack of confidence are holding you back from becoming this man?

_____

_____

_____

_____

_____

_____

_____

_____

_____

_____

_____

_____

_____

_____

_____

"Motivation is what gets you started. Habit is what keeps you going"

Jim Ryun

Chapter 3

Habits by Addition

We all have habits -- the good, the bad, and the ugly. So how do you go about breaking a bad habit? I'm talking the ones that hold you back, push you farther from your goals, and may even hurt the ones you love?

I have an excellent plan that has been highly successful in my life. And here's the secret -- it's not just about removing a habit, it's about adding a new one.

I'm going to tell you my story of chewing, and how I successfully quit a 26-year habit on my own. Although my method was simple, it involved daily choices on my part, and I managed to not only drop my chewing habit, but also add in healthier ones that helped me be the man I wanted to be.

I started chewing at 14 years old. I did this because growing up, my dad chewed too. I remember watching him and thinking it was cool, so I tried my first at about 7 or 8 years old. Of course, it didn't go well -- I got buzzed, threw up, and thought I was going to pass out.

Unfortunately, I didn't let it stop me from trying it again and again.

I got to the point to where I started chewing all the time. By the time I was 16, I was chewing *a can a day*. This went on for a long time, and I tried to quit six times in total, and used gum, patches, and medication, but nothing worked.

When I attended Warrior Week and learned about the 90-day outcomes, it changed everything. Although I had my goals and targets set, I never considered establishing a goal about chewing.

One day in February 2016, while in my office at work, this sort of voice came to me and asked, "What if you could just stop chewing until your next chew? What would happen if you did that? If you craved one, you did 20 pushups instead of the chew? And at that point, if you still wanted it, you could have one."

So for this one particular day, as soon as I craved a chew, I did 20 pushups. To my surprise, it took away the first craving. But then 30 minutes to an hour later, it happened again. For the first two days *I did 400-500 pushups a day*. I was like, "Holy shit -- what's going on? I crave this all day!" I was chewing every day at work while training clients, but no one knew; it was something I hid. My wife knew about my habit, but she didn't really care.

I realized after a week of following this new plan of habits by addition, I went from 400-500 pushups a day to just 200-300. Every time I wanted a chew, I was lying to myself about how I felt, and worse -- I was lying to other people. My realization was that I would get triggered or pissed off by someone, and it was *easier to put a chew in than to actually deal with the real issue.* So basically, every single time I wanted a chew, I was lying to myself about how I felt. It always started with me.

My inner voice was starting to speak to me, "I'm a fitness professional and am teaching people how to be healthy, yet I have this hidden secret of addiction that is weighing on my conscience." The integrity (that I take a lot of pride in) was just not there. Sure, on the outside I was healthy to the average person, but on the inside, I had an addiction and was going through a can of tobacco every day.

Instead of focusing on *taking away* chew, I focused on *adding in a habit* that could replace it. This can be correlated to many different addictions and habits. For example, if you want to quit eating candy, instead of taking away food, start doing pushups every time you crave a sweet. Or, if every time you want a cigarette, you walk around the outside of your house instead.

You can realistically stop anything by focusing on something you can do instead. As soon as you want something that might hurt you or your mission, replace it with something that serves you. It distracts your mind and it gets you what you *really* want.

Does it work? I am proud to report that I haven't had any chew since that day. It took me about 3.5 weeks to fully quit. Did I crave it? Yes, but the signal in my mind was, "Dude, you're lying if you crave it." I shifted my mindset and asked, "What am I lying about? What's the truth in this? What do I need to fix or who do I need to talk to fix this?" Instead of me putting in a chew in and saying, "Well that doesn't really matter," I would confront a person and say, "Hey, this upset me or pissed me off."

Addiction is a crutch, a distraction, an escape. I had a 26-year habit of lying. A 26-year habit of not facing reality. I see this all the time where people say, "I just can't break this habit," but the problem is they don't want to deal with reality. **The lie is easier than telling the truth**.

After the push-ups were added in, I switched those out for conversation. When I felt like I needed a chew, I would throw myself into conversation to deal with the issue. I then leveraged this skill of facing the truth into other areas of my life.

Let's take another example. Every morning I got into the habit of checking my cell phone first thing. This led to me wasting 1.5 hours at the start of every day instead of being present and productive. Instead, I immediately got out of bed, had a green drink and read. I would focus on my Core-4 daily habits and would not look at my phone until I was done.

Typically, you'll watch people in this cycle, they'll take away a habit and replace it with something just as bad. They'll trick their mind into thinking, "Hey this is better," but it isn't because they're still in the habit loop.

Have you found yourself in this place?

If instead, you add a positive habit to take away a bad habit, you'll find that you're actually moving toward your results at a rapid pace. Dependency is a crutch and makes you weaker by nature, so when you remove dependencies, you instantly become stronger.

I had zero desire that day to quit chewing -- I just had a desire to *quit until the next craving.* When you're setting big goals, even your 90-day goals, sometimes it's most effective to break it down, choice by choice, step by step.

Keep putting one foot in the other and it's going to propel you forward to becoming your best self.

CHALLENGE YOURSELF

What are you addicted to? Is it social media, food, alcohol, cigarettes? Identify one of these baits in your life that you want to change and then identify the habit that you want to replace it with. Make it a measurable habit (such as push-ups, squats, adding a serving of vegetables, walking around a building, etc.), and test it for a week. Ask yourself, "Am I going to continue this bad habit or replace it with a healthy one?"

_____

_____

_____

_____

_____

_____

_____

_____

_____

"We gain the strength of the temptation we resist."

Ralph Waldo Emerson

Chapter 4

When You Want to Quit, You're Only 40% There

Have you ever given up on something? Have you ever felt, "I've done enough," so you quit, only to feel disappointed later for not pushing yourself harder?

I want you to know something. When you quit, you're only quitting on yourself.

I'm not perfect, I've been there too. I've put myself in situations where I absolutely wanted to quit, but did I?

I'd like to tell you the story of the time I spent six months training for Kokoro, a U.S. Navy SEAL training program that's open to civilians.

When I arrived at the training ground in Temecula, CA, it was a sweltering 112 degrees F. That, right there, is almost enough to make you want to quit before you start.

I knew that this program would be intense and would challenge me to my core, but I had no idea that it would be so insanely difficult right from the start. To kick off this 53-hour-straight program, we had to do a physical training test to gain entry. We went to the tennis court where they had us drop down and do bear crawls.

Have you ever touched a tennis court on a 112-degree day? In the first activity alone, our hands got completely burned off. For the remainder of the day, anything we did was with injured, split-open hands.

The SEALS led us in a workout called Murph which involved running one mile, performing 300 squats, 200 sit-ups, 100 pull ups, and a mile-long run on the back side. If this wasn't tough enough, you had to wear a weighted backpack and carry an eight-pound weapon. We were given one hour and 10 minutes to complete the physical challenge.

I had the thought of quitting during Kokoro, and asked myself, "What am I giving up if I quit?" My answer? The commitment I made to myself.

Inside of this, another challenger and I were the first to come through. I wanted to quit and then I saw other guys come in worse. I'm talking they were getting thrown in ice baths for 45 minutes just to revive them and bring them back to life.

When I wanted to quit, I couldn't help but think of the words of Mark Divine from *Unbeatable Minds.* He states that *if you feel like quitting, you're only at 40% capacity and still have another 60% left.*

As I began to see other people come in, I reminded myself, "Dude I'm only at 40%." At that moment, I began to shift, and I started to cheer other guys on. I realized that if this is it and I made it through, then I can handle anything in life beyond this. I still have 60% in the tank, and it was a complete mind shift.

Over the next two days, I kept reminding myself that I was only at 40%. It was a lesson that I continued to remind myself of for 53 straight hours. I'm telling you, it was not easy -- there was no sleep, we were dehydrated, we were fed, but we got our asses kicked for three days straight. We started with 18 guys and only 11 finished.

After this test of my will and endurance, I realized that I could apply this thinking to anything. No matter how hard you're working in business, or in marriage, no matter how bad it seems, there is still 60% more room for improvement. Even inside prayer and meditation, there is still so much more room for growth.

The message I want to impart to you is that whether things in your life are going great or not, you still have plenty left. You're not even close to your capacity.

Giving up is always there when the stakes are high, but whether you go through it or not is what's going to separate you. If you're going to break your promise to yourself, then you're going to break your promise to someone else. If I can't keep my commitments with myself, it will be *impossible* to keep them with anybody else.

What we do matters most in this, if we take the easy road now, we might do it somewhere else down the road.

I remember while training, I'd think, "I'm just going to run this far, it's enough." And then "Nope, I'm going to run another mile just for *thinking* about quitting." or I'd make myself do 10 more reps just for thinking of quitting.

Just like in my last chapter, I was taking a bad habit (considering quitting) and replacing it with a good habit (pushing myself harder).

After I completed the Kokoro challenge, I debated whether to do another physical challenge and continue to beat up my body, or instead, leverage my success from Kokoro into another area in my life. I realized that there's a Kokoro inside my Being, Balance, Body, and Business, and I need to incorporate it into that instead of going through another physical challenge.

Have I ever quit something that was important to me? Yes. I gave up college football in 1996. The entire reason I even wanted to go to college was to play football, and I quit because I had a son at the time. Although I gave up on my dream with good reason, I learned something from taking a different direction in my life. I regretted quitting at the time, but now I don't. I will admit though, that in my mind, it still stings a little to say that I gave up on my dream.

I challenge you to empower yourself. Believe in yourself and follow through on your dreams, vision and goals, no matter how difficult. Remember, when you want to quit, you're only at 40% and you still have another 60% to push with. Your tank is never as empty as it appears.

CHALLENGE YOURSELF

Take an amazing experience that you've had and write it out. Now leverage the lesson from this experience and apply it to another area of your life. Is there something you have given up on in your life? Do you regret it? What have you learned from it?

_____

_____

_____

_____

_____

_____

_____

_____

_____

_____

_____

_____

"Never give up, for that is just the place and time that the tide will turn."

Harriet Beecher Stowe

Chapter 5

You Can Do Anything You Put Your Mind To

Have you ever accomplished something massive and when you look back on it after the fact, you think, "Why did I doubt myself? I was *more* than capable."

In my last chapter, I spoke about the importance of not quitting, and the next level of that is accelerating even beyond your current goals and on to something bigger.

Have you ever participated in a Tough Mudder event? It's a several-mile loop complete with obstacles to demonstrate to yourself and teammates how badass you are. Tough Mudder isn't about racing others or racing against the clock, instead it's about pushing yourself to discover what you're really made of.

I signed up for the World's Toughest Mudder, a 24-hour around-the-clock version of the classic Tough Mudder. When I decided to do this, it was four months out. I let a couple months go by without training, even though I made this commitment of completing 50 miles. At that point, the longest I had ever run was 8-9 miles, so it was a lofty goal.

I recall that I was super busy at the time, coaching and doing a lot with my business. As a result, I had stopped running and wasn't even sure if I could run five miles, let alone 50. Before I knew it, I found myself 6-8 weeks out from the event, running a mile a day to work back into it. I remember thinking 24 hours prior, "Oh shit, I committed to 50 miles and I don't know how I'm going to pull this off."

The day of the event arrived. Each lap around World's Toughest Mudder course was five miles long. After the first lap, I thought, "Shit this isn't too bad." After lap one, they opened up the obstacles for every round after that.

A detail that I forgot to share was that I went into this with a fracture in my hand. Two weeks prior, I screwed my hand up, and had to wear a hard cast on my arm during the event. This meant that I couldn't pull up with one side and had to use one arm for everything on the course.

Once I hit my third lap I felt like shit, so I paced off and went back to my tent. I sat there, thinking to myself, "I've already done more than I've ever done in my life, so I can just be done."

Have you ever said that to yourself?

Luckily, I came around and I thought, "No, I can go to 25 miles. I can do this." I began to coach myself every time I felt doubt creep in. I was alone in my own experience, talking myself through each lap. "Now you're at 15, want to go again?" or "I wonder if I could go through another lap?"

I want to make it clear that some of these laps took a very long time to complete. My first lap took about a 1 hour, and by the end, each lap took about 2 hours and 30 minutes to complete.

Halfway through, on mile 25, it was 9 or 10 p.m. at night. I remember that the sun was down, and it began to get cold. Doubt set in with each and every lap, as I had been at it for hours.

I told myself, "Okay, I'm going to challenge myself every mile." So I began to just talk myself through every lap and every obstacle, and did it in my head, out loud, or both.

At midnight they opened up a 35-foot cliff, so that when you finished your lap, you would step on a platform and drop 35 feet, then swim and climb up some rocks. This would signify the end of your lap and you'd be done.

I think I made it to 30 or 35 miles, but by the time I was done, it was 3 a.m., so I slept a couple hours, woke up and did it again. At that point, everything in my body ached and hurt, but I started my next lap.

Negative self-talk kicked in again, and I thought, "You've already done more than you've ever done and now you're in a double marathon." I was about to start my 45th mile and I wanted to give up, but at mile 50 I knew I'd receive a patch. I was so close and let this award incentivize me.

I was on my last lap and I wanted to quit but talked myself out of it at every obstacle. I realized I practically had zero training leading up to the World's Toughest Mudder and *it made me realize how far I can push my mind in any situation*. I trained while running 4-6 miles at a time and was now running 50 miles!

So I finished the lap, everybody was cheering, and we jumped off the cliff. I got in, received my patch and I realized that I miscounted -- I actually did 55 miles!

That night after the event, I got a massage and just the sensation of the lady touching my leg nearly sent me off the table. It took me six weeks to recover from the World's Toughest Mudder. It was the worst pain of my life, but the experience taught me a valuable lesson. I realized that *I had the power of my mind to talk myself in or out of anything*.

I can tell you I wanted to quit 100 times and talked myself out of it every time.

I wanted to quit because I was doing something I was completely unfamiliar with, but I always like to challenge myself. Every single lap, I challenged myself to beat my previous one.

No matter what, you can convince yourself to keep fighting that extra day. It was the belief in myself that I can do anything that I'm committed to, even if it seems impossible at the time, that pushed me through. ***Every lap went from being impossible to being more than possible***.

I want you to know that it's all in the power of the mind. You're able to do anything, if you just convince your mind.

CHALLENGE YOURSELF

What limitations have you put on yourself? Your body? Your being? Your balance? Your business? What is one thing you have always wanted to do that challenges your comfort zone? Why aren't you doing it? What's stopping you from doing it? Today I challenge you to pull out your credit card and commit to doing one thing that scares you?

_____

_____

_____

_____

_____

_____

_____

_____

_____

_____

"Whether you think you can, or you think you can't -- you're right."

Henry Ford

Chapter 6

Setting the Tone

I want you to realize that you are in control of more than you know. That your life doesn't have to happen *to* you, that it can happen *because of* you? That it can even happen *for* you.

Every day when you wake up, you have the new opportunity to set your intention for the day to set the tone for how you handle yourself, your business and your interactions with those around you.

One year ago, I began living my life with setting a daily intention. Each morning I would wake up and would set the tone for my day. I started my practice of setting an intention with the first goal of selling my business.

For almost 12 years, I owned my own fitness training businesses, but got to the point where I was burnt out, bored and wanted a change of identity. I wanted to be known as someone who was more than just the guy who does fitness. It felt very one-dimensional and I wanted to shift my life focus.

Each morning I would take 5-10 minutes to write out my intention of the day. As an example, I stated that I wanted to sell my business by June 30, 2018. This was an intention that I started setting six months prior, in December of 2017. I started reading this intention every day, and deliberately took control of what I wanted to do and who I wanted to become.

I then broke my target into a short-term outcome. My mission became, "What do I want to accomplish and pull off *today?*" Who do I have to become to sell my business?

I would meditate on my intention of cutting the cord with my business. I truly wanted a new purpose in life and this was my first step. I think that the hardest thing for me was having no idea of how the hell I was going to sell my business in the beginning. In all honesty, I didn't even know if I could pull it off. Putting my intention down on paper and reminding myself that I was putting energy into figuring out how to sell it, made me make the commitment to selling it.

For the next two months, I didn't do anything active towards my goal. I finally decided to find a broker, and we went through a six-week-long process. They organized the paperwork to sell my business and had the entire package set up for me. It was a multi-million dollar deal involving two training facilities that were doing almost $2 million a year in revenue. Although it was a healthy business and I was making great money, I was simply burnt out and bored. It was time.

Buying and selling a training business is different than a gym. You have a certain number of members with a gym, and it's just paper. With selling a training facility, you have people attached to you and to your trainers, so it is a little different and tricky, plus I had to keep quiet about selling it.

Would you believe, that once it launched, we had had a full-price offer in just three days?

The week before my business was set to close, my buyer found out his wife had rectal cancer. He contacted me and said, "The good news is that I have everything ready to go to close on the sale of your business, but the bad news is that we don't know how severe the cancer is. We will find out this week." He called me back that Wednesday, and said, "My wife has a four- to six-month recovery period, and I need to be by her side the whole time. I'm not sure if buying the business is the right thing for me right now."

I talked it over with my wife and we were in agreement. I contacted the buyer and said, "The number one thing you need to do is focus on your wife right now."

The deal was off, but I believe it was for good reason with something better in store.

You see, I had a manager who worked for me for over 11 years, managing my business, and before that, we worked together for five years in a different gym. I asked my broker what it would take to just sell my business to my manager. He came up with a plan, I made an offer to my manager, and he agreed. Had I known he wanted it, I would have gone straight to my manager in the first place, but I didn't know if he would have been in that place at that time.

We spent the next couple months working with it, and the final sale closed on August 30th of this year. I went from saying "I will sell Innovative Fitness by June 30, 2018," to having my manager agree to the sale on July 1 -- it was right around my target date June 30th after all.

This all started as an idea, an intention. It was just one of those things where I don't know if in the beginning I actually believed the intention, but *from doing it every day, I basically called this forward*.

When you write down your intentions and speak about them, you're putting energy into them and calling them forward. When you put something out there, you're going to get something back. Although there's always doubt and fear of, "What if I can't do this," or "What if I fail?" Instead, I suggest that you just call it forward, shift your focus, and make your intention your top-of-mind awareness. That way, when an opportunity comes up, you can jump on it right away.

I began setting intentions across all areas of my life. My intention could be a workout for that day, a business goal for that day, or being vulnerable about something and sharing it with my wife, children or business partner. I had to do this with my manager when I said, "Hey man, I had this business sold a week ago, found out about the cancer, and I want to see if you want it. I believe that this was the way it was supposed to happen and that you are the guy who is supposed to buy this."

So I made the goal to start each morning with writing down and saying my intention out loud 3-5 times a day. I set a hard date and something I could shoot for and measure, and I think that's a crucial piece.

Today, I can think about where I was a year ago. I was coaching clients, had two businesses, and was living in Washington state. Today I live in Southern California with my wife and kids, I work full-time for Wake Up Warrior, and have no gym businesses. Setting that intention over the last year got me where I am today.

This super powerful practice instills belief in myself and calls things forward that aren't yet there, but soon will be. Think of it as awakening the universe -- if you don't talk, think or speak about it, how does the universe even know?

I want you to add this daily practice into your life. Set your intentions every day to have more control over your life and drive it in the direction you want it to go. Everybody makes list of things *to do,* not of things they *want.* I encourage you to

make a list of things you want, not of things to do. Be prepared to watch your life change before your very eyes.

CHALLENGE YOURSELF

Write down one intention for each of the four areas of your life and then start speaking it out loud three to five times each day. If you feel doubt in any situation, just speak it out. Write down your daily intentions every morning, recognizing that they can change every day, and know they don't always have to be the same. Write it down enough to memorize it, stating, "My intention today is ___."

_____

_____

_____

_____

_____

_____

_____

_____

_____

_____

"Attitude is a choice. Happiness is a choice. Optimism is a choice. Kindness is a choice. Giving is a choice. Respect is a choice. Whatever choice you make makes you. Choose wisely."

Roy T. Bennett

Chapter 7

Blaming My Father

At what point do you stop placing blame on others, forgive them, and take accountability for your own feelings, choices, and actions? As they say, holding onto anger is like drinking poison and expecting the other person to die.

For those of you who grew up with an alcoholic parent, this story may resonate. For those of you who have a strained relationship with your parent(s), this story may also resonate. Either way, I want to tell you about my tumultuous relationship with my alcoholic father and how I got over it.

For as long as I can remember, my dad was an alcoholic. At the age of five or six, I began to witness my dad's daily habit. He would come home from work and immediately start drinking beer. If that wasn't enough, he involved me in his addiction. I so clearly remember having to run downstairs every 30 minutes to replenish his supply. He had a dingy fridge that kept all his beer, and I remember this fridge because it had a certain smell to it. I had to grab one Old Milwaukee Light or Heidelberg after the other and deliver them on repeat to my dad upstairs. The cycle would repeat every 30 minutes from the moment he got home to the time he went to bed.

My dad was the most intimidating man I knew. When he came home, I remember feeling scared and tried to read which version of my dad came home. Was he going to be super nice? Or was he going to be angry, pissed off, and out of control? Most of the time, it seemed like he was always angry.

My dad was always consistent with anything he did. My parents would show up to every sport and every game that we had. My dad would come to baseball games in the summer, with a cooler of beer, drinking during the game, and getting in fights with parents on the other team.

It seemed like everybody drank back then and there was always chaos, and there was always something to be pissed and angry about.

I remember lots of verbal abuse growing up. My dad would frequently argue and fight with my mom and my brother, and it would often get physical. Funny enough, I could handle the physical stuff -- it was the mental abuse that was hard to handle.

I remember being a kid and my dad calling me a pussy if I cried. When you're a kid with big emotions and difficult situations, and your dad calls you a pussy for crying, it beats you down. I remember that sticking with me for a long time.

I was grateful that through sports like boxing or football, I could take out my frustration in a safe place. I used athletics to release my pent-up anger and rage toward my dad and was grateful to have sports as my outlet. I even remember the point that my dad started liking boxing more than I did. It's because he criticized me in the ring asking, "Why didn't you do this or that?" It made me resent boxing and I hated it for a while.

My dad was a hard-working blue-collar type. He was a butcher until I was age 10, then he did concrete work through my high school years, and then became a mechanic. One thing about my dad is that he was always working. He was from Montana and had a strong work ethic and a kind of hardcore redneck personality.

I lived at home with my parents until I was 18 and moved out just two months before graduating high school.

When I say that my dad was intimidating, it wasn't just because of his anger, it was also because of his athleticism. In his youth, he was a badass high school football player and wrestled in college at Washington State University.

I remember the day that I actually beat him in wrestling for the first time. We were wrestling, and I went toe-to-toe with him, and he couldn't take me down. In that moment, my dad accepted me as a man and there was no more intimidation.

I moved out a few months before high school graduation, then moved to Santa Maria, California, for junior college to play football. That lasted only one Semester. Unfortunately, my time there was cut short because I found out my girlfriend was pregnant. She was a senior in high school and lived back in Spokane, Washington. I made the choice to move back home and back in with my parents. Shortly after my Son Taylor was born, he and his mother (my girlfriend at the time), moved in with me at my parents' house.

It was a bit surreal because so much had happened and changed in my life, and when I moved back home, it was exactly the same. Dad was drinking, angry, and fighting, and always having issues with me and my mom. Eventually, my son and his mom moved out.

I then started a cycle of moving in and out of my parents' house for about two to three years. My dad finally quit drinking around the time I was 25 or 26, and he gave it up for ten whole years. Although this was a great development, we kind of grew apart and didn't talk for a while.

I needed a change and moved to Seattle, where I ended up working in gyms. I moved because my son and his mother left to live in Utah, and I needed to have a fresh start. After my ex left, I was in and out of jail and I got in a lot of trouble. I always

MAN IN THE MIRROR

felt like my parents blamed me for all of that and they were disappointed in me. I carried around a lot of shame and guilt for that.

I felt that if I had a father who showed up for me, I would have turned out differently. I was blaming someone else and not taking personal accountability for my own choices and actions.

The last time I moved out, it was pretty troublesome. My parents caught me with $15k dollars in steroids that I was selling at the time, so it wasn't like I was some class A citizen. I remember my parents saying, "You're not going to come back this time." So I just kind of left and never came back. I didn't go back home for over a year. I moved to Seattle to get away from everything. I moved with a box of clothes and some photos, I didn't even have a car, I literally had nothing.

When I met my wife Katie a few years later, everything changed. We started having kids and my parents came around more. When my son and daughter were ages 8 and 5, they went to stay with my parents for a week in Spokane, WA. Katie and I made the drive to pick them back up, and during this time, I was preparing to go to Warrior Week for a second time that year.

Because of this, I was ready to go to my parents and finally have a deep conversation with my dad, so that we could strengthen our relationship. When we arrived, my wife noticed that my dad seemed kind of weird. I was on edge and noticed something was up too, but I didn't know what it was. Dad started making inappropriate comments and then got pissed at my son for crying, of all things. I was immediately triggered. My wife said to me, "I think he's drinking again."

I pulled my mom aside to find out what was going on. At first she lied to me, but then finally confessed, "He's actually been drinking for the past six months." I lost my shit and said, "That's bullshit! Why would you lie about this? You lied when I was a kid and now you're lying again, and this is just is bad."

Angrily, I confronted my dad outside and asked, "When the fuck did you start drinking again?" He got pissed off and yelled back at me, so I challenged, "Hit me! If you want to hit me, hit me! I can tell you this, I will never come here again, and my kids will never come here again if you do this. I grew up with this and I'm not going to deal with it in my thirties, and I am definitely not going to put my wife and kids through this!"

What happened next was unexpected.

My dad, who was shitfaced and beet red, started crying. I realized that he carried around all this guilt and shame for so long. My dad's dad was never around, was terrible, was super angry, and always pissed off. In my dad's eyes, he was better than his own father, so he didn't realize what he was doing to us. He saw it as he was doing better job and was not emulating his father. He always had this guilt and shame from drinking, and I began to realize that he didn't know any different. *He only knew what he knew.*

I coached my dad out of his pain and his pit and I forgave him for everything that he did to me as a kid. I felt like I was the parent, I was able to release his pain, and in return, it released mine.

I realized in that moment, that my dad did the best that he could with the tools that he had. By forgiving him, he was able to forgive himself. **He stopped drinking the next day** and I don't think he's had a drink since. My mom said if I hadn't done that they wouldn't have stayed married.

When you coach your parents it's like "Holy shit, I don't know what's happening." You hit that realization of, "Oh my god, my parents aren't really equipped with the tools I have."

Boys are usually affected most by their fathers and girls, by their mothers. There is a deep pain inside a lot of men today from their fathers. I played the victim for a long time and blamed my dad for so much.

I always looked up to my dad growing up. Like I said, he was the most intimidating man I knew and all I ever wanted from my dad was love. Unfortunately, I never got that as a kid growing up. Instead, if I showed any emotion, he would get mad and insult me, so I always wanted more from him, but I never got it.

A lot of guys carry around this pain of how their dads showed up or didn't. As a reminder, our dads learned from their fathers and they did the best they could.

My dad did bring some positives to my life. He taught me how to work hard and taught me about things like commitment. He was always up early, no matter what. Even if he drank, he was still up at 4 a.m. working on something. I don't know anybody who worked harder than my dad.

He also showed up to any sport I was playing and coached me when I was younger. He wasn't disconnected, you just didn't get a whole lot of love. It seems to be the norm for his generation, and for the one before that. He taught me about sports, working on cars, and doing handy work, so I was constantly learning from my dad.

Our relationship was painful up until age 36. Once I forgave him and tried to understand him, it helped us both move forward. Today we have moved on from any negativity in our past.

Realizing that I was in control of my life, in control of my reactions, and that I could set daily intentions and habits, was not only empowering, it was also freeing. Learning that I was better equipped with tools than my own father, I was able to coach him, help him, and forgive him.

Are you holding on to pain from the past? Are you ready to build your inner strength, set challenges for yourself, reach goals, achieve calm, and forgive? There is no day like today to start.

CHALLENGE YOURSELF

Think about your mom and dad and go back to the #1 pain that you remember as a child. Now, simply write out everything you remember and send them a message that you forgive them. By forgiving them, you're forgiving yourself too. It's time to heal.

_____

_____

_____

_____

_____

_____

_____

_____

_____

_____

_____

_____

"The weak can never forgive. Forgiveness is the attribute of the strong."

Mahatma Gandhi

Chapter 8

The Impossible Game

I am a firm believer that you can do anything you set your mind to. You can start planning and setting intentions today to become a stronger, happier, healthier version of yourself within the next 90 days. All it takes is getting your heart and head in the game, and if you consistently keep it up, and continue gaining momentum, you'll hit some massive targets by next year. You will love who you see in the mirror -- the ultimate version of you.

The key to this maximum level of happiness is a challenge-based lifestyle.

As a disciplined athlete and someone who loves competition, I always created challenges for my body in a push to be the best. Although I was mostly consistent with it throughout my life, there was a time that I shut it down for a while.

The moment I decided to stop playing football and leave my junior college once my son was born, was the first big break from a challenge. Needing something else, I got into bodybuilding for about five or six years but shut that down to go into work mode. As a trainer, I focused primarily on work and working out. During this time, I got married and had kids, and that life change really shut down my physical goals. I pushed aside lifelong practices and could feel the difference.

When I did my first Warrior Week in 2016, it was also my first introduction to 90-day challenges. I hadn't been super focused on working out in a long time and the challenges began to change my body.

Although I was a trainer and wasn't in terrible shape, I wasn't in good shape by my standards.

What did my first 90 day challenge do for me? I lost 7-8% body fat, went to running a 12K after not running at all, and my marriage improved. I changed my lifestyle, and whatever I committed to, I was *always* successful at it. I wanted to be the best at whatever I did.

As a trainer, I'd ask, "Who is the best trainer?" From there, I would learn from that individual, go to classes, and become the best, so that there was no question in my mind.

As I began to do these challenges, I took my kids and wife on dates and I experienced massive growth. After each 90-day period, I would start a new challenge, and this transitioned into living a challenge-based lifestyle. ***Every 90 days I did something that felt impossible at the beginning.*** And you know what happened? Every day or week that I stuck with it, it seemed more possible. Every three months, I asked myself, "Hey, what do I want to accomplish in the next 90 days? Who would I have to become to pull this off? I accomplished a goal with running but *now* what can I do?" I never stopped in my commitment to growth.

I began to break down every area of my life and do all four areas -- Body, Being, Balance and Business -- every 90 days, not just one area as I had gotten accustomed to in the past. This involved more than just a physical challenge.

For example, I would go to church 12 times over 12 weeks and journaled what I got out of it. Another target was to shoot a video every day for 90 days and put it on social media. (At that time, I hated doing videos and so that was a big deal.) And I remember instead of making 90 videos, I kept going and shot 115! Then when I did Warrior Week again, I began my own coaching program, called Project Alpha. It has been my pride and pleasure to introduce this concept with other men at my gym. This took off into me wanting to do this full-time as a coach.

These 90-day challenges brought me back to my roots, and back to who I was at the core. When I was in sports, I did two workouts a day, and by high school I was the strongest kid in my school.

Once again, I was willing to do whatever it took to be the best.

What the challenge-based lifestyle and these 90-day challenges sparked in me was that purpose to be the best again, and not in just one area. I wanted to be the best in Warrior, and to say to myself, "Hey dude, these challenges will seem impossible, but I'm going to do this."

I think now I am on my 16th or 17th challenge. I feel like I went from 90-day challenges to mastering the art and science of actually creating and executing a challenge. It takes a level of mastery to be able to identify what I want and who I would have to become over the next 90 days or next year and then break that down into a 90-day segment. It's important to have something to stick to, and to challenge yourself in small, measurable, incremental steps.

Some people say it takes 67 days to create a habit. I think it takes one day, done 67 times to create a habit. I talked to you about this -- when I asked myself, "What if I could just stop chewing until the next time I wanted to chew?' I focused on my choices over one day, versus setting a larger goal of quitting within 90 days. It is okay to start in incremental steps, because with consistency, they will add up.

Here's the thing, the big picture doesn't matter if I haven't done what I need to today. We *underestimate* what we can do in 90 days or a year, and we *overestimate* what we can do in a day or a week. That's what stops us from accomplishing what we want.

Switching challenges every quarter makes sense. Most people get bored 8-12 weeks in with what they're doing, and it becomes easy to lose interest and momentum. If you change up what you're doing, and reset your outcomes every 12 weeks, it's a recipe for success that will continue to propel you forward.

An important component is to emphasize all four areas with each challenge, but they don't have to be huge outcomes in all four areas. For example, my first physical challenge was dropping 7-8% body fat and going from not running to running a 12K (which I ended up doing in only 45 days). My next one was a workout called Fight Gone Bad for CrossFit and I wanted to beat the record at Warrior Week. My next challenge was Krav Maga level 1 test, and after that I continued with levels 2 and 3. I then challenged myself to get into SEAL Fit 20x, then to Kokoro, and then to level 4 and 5 in Krav Maga.

But these physical challenges are just scratching the surface.

I quit chewing, and that was a huge goal. After stopping that habit, I had my teeth cleaned and fixed. I quit eating red meat for 90 days, I took meditation classes, and I even met with a psychic for energy work. This was an incredible experience that lasted for 18 months total, and she became a coach to me. The energy work with her opened me up to God, more than anything else. I'll admit, at first I thought I was going to go to Hell for seeing her, but know I know that psychic readers simply read your energy and chakras -- that shit's no joke.

Some examples of my business challenges were earning $50k in 90 days or $150k in 90 days, and then I take those earnings home and put them into my "creating a legacy" account. Another important target was learning how to create marketing strategies with landing pages, and funnels for advertising on social media. I remember going from investing $5-$7k in Facebook ads and getting a couple hundred thousand out of it back three or four years ago before everyone started doing it.

My business goals were always about creating something new. I'd assess what was one new thing I wanted to create in my business and what was something else that I could repackage. It is constantly a flow of something new and something repackaged.

When I examined why I wanted to undergo these challenges and improve, I realized that my true source of strength and purpose was my family. As part of my Balance challenges, I took my kids on dates, took my wife on dates and trips, long weekends, and more vacations. We went from one vacation a year to two family vacations and two long weekends just for us. We just started doing more stuff together. I also wrote my wife a book with affirmations, and for our 10-year anniversary, I gave her a bigger diamond.

I want to see just how much you can accomplish with a challenge-based lifestyle. You'll break down what you want to achieve in all four areas of your life and reset with new goals every 90 days.

When you create a game you can play every 90 days, you will go from the impossible to the possible. It will lead to you the person you want to become, year after year. It's all about committing to a challenge mindset and a growth mindset.

This is what a challenge-based lifestyle is all about. Are you ready to get in the game?

CHALLENGE YOURSELF

Sit down and get clear on what you want over the next 90 days and ask why you want it. How will you pull it off? What skills do you have and what mindset will you need to pull it off? Who you will you have to become to pull this off? Once you've done this, go to your habits and line them up with your outcomes to make sure they are in alignment. Once you start doing these 90-day challenges, you will find that they will set you up with where you want to be next year.

_____

_____

_____

_____

_____

_____

_____

_____

_____

"A champion shows who he is by what he does."

Evander Holyfield

Chapter 9

Calm and Suppression

Have you ever tried to act a certain way, and maintain the facade no matter how you felt? Have you put up a front while you were scared, sad, angry, or lonely? What did that do to you? Did it manifest in other ways?

I want to tell you about my journey in learning when to show and when to control my emotions. This is a result of a couple of unfortunate events that taught me who I was and how I both handled (and mishandled) things.

I had a son at a very early age, 19, and during that time I found myself in and out of trouble. I was on tons of steroids and pain pills and was selling them along with other drugs. My son, his mother, and I, were living with my parents. My father's alcoholism and anger issues were still present, and inevitably, my relationship with my son's mother deteriorated.

My ex was in the process of moving out with my son when we got into an argument one day. I asked her to please let my mom watch our son instead of taking him to daycare, but she refused, so the conversation got heated. As this was happening, her new boyfriend was watching this all go down from inside his car.

The situation escalated and when she swung to hit me, I put my arm up to block it. I was a trained boxer, after all, and I knew how to guard myself from a hit. Unfortunately, when I did this, and she fell backwards, got up, and ran to the car. I was so enraged that she was acting like this, so I went to the car and started banging on the window. I challenged her boyfriend. "Get the fuck out of the car so I can beat the shit of you," I yelled. Of course, he didn't want to stand up to me and they drove off.

It took me a while to calm down, and I headed into work for the day. When I returned home, I took a shower, and while in there, I heard something outside my window. I put on a towel and when I looked outside, and I saw a cop. With his gun drawn he asked, "Are you Jesse Ewell? I need you to come outside."

Not sure what this was all about, I threw on some shorts with no shirt and stepped outside. Here I was, this massive guy at 250 lbs., and I was quickly rushed and taken down to the ground. I was completely caught off-guard.

The cops arrested me, saying that I hit my ex and that her boyfriend was a witness. I was taken to jail and spent a day there, on charges of domestic violence and assault.

When I went to court, I got the charges reduced on the condition that I go to domestic violence counseling. This entire situation infuriated me because I had to go in and say, "I beat my ex-girlfriend." You can't say, "I didn't really hit her. She hit me, and I blocked it." Nope. Instead you have to play their game. It's almost like going to AA and saying, "I drank once, I got caught and now have to call myself an alcoholic." That won't fly.

To make matters worse, because of court orders, I had to go through regular drug testing for the next year. They found some steroids in my son's diaper bag that I had forgot to take out. So every week, I had to do a drug and alcohol test. I had to call in every day and if my color came up, I had to immediately go down and take a test for a full year.

The story doesn't stop there, unfortunately. I moved out, got a roommate, and 18 months went by. My roommate and I got into a fight because he stole some drugs from me, so I ended up punching him in the eye. It swelled up and looked like a softball was attached to the side of his head. When the cops arrived they said, "You're on domestic violence probation, and for beating up your roommate, you're coming to jail." Because we lived together this classified as a domestic dispute.

Yet again, I was charged with domestic violence and had to attend domestic violence counseling. So here I was, at 20 or 21 years old, with this agreement and four years' probation, otherwise I would go to jail.

I plead guilty to a misdemeanor and received a deferred sentence. As long as I didn't do anything for four years, no charges would be brought up against me, and these would be dropped.

Although not the best of experiences, I learned some odd takeaways from all the domestic violence counseling and anger management. They always taught that you have to be calm, suppress your feelings and that you can never lose control. Society doesn't want you to express your feelings or emotions and so you're taught to hide them.

They'll tell you, "Don't be angry or mad," but what happens when you bottle it all up inside? When you don't have a release, you end up holding onto it all the time. A huge part of it is that I held onto it already as a kid, because my dad would criticize me any time I showed emotions. This counseling almost made it worse, because **now I was bottling it all up and it was killing who I was**.

What they taught in counseling made me believe that I couldn't be who I wanted to be because people couldn't handle that side of me. I was always angry, but not really sure why, and I was always stuffing it in.

At least when I was in football or boxing I could put on a mask, be me, and let it out in a safe place. When I didn't have that outlet anymore, I didn't have anywhere to release it, so I'd hold it in until it blew up.

I have since learned from Warrior, that people *can* handle that part of me and I don't always have to be calm and suppress my emotions. Energy is huge for me, and when it is suppressed, you can't express who you are or how you feel. This was one reason that I sold my gym, because in the last two years of ownership, it no longer made my heart rate fly up. I just felt like I couldn't be myself in that environment anymore.

If you ever feel this way, you have to make a change. If you can't be *all of you* and have people accept all of you, then you're in the wrong environment. You're going to have to make changes, so you don't suppress who you are.

These suppressions lead to numbing and sedating with things like drugs, alcohol, porn, TV, or gaming. The people who do this, they basically go to sleep. They're alive but they go to sleep. They are the people who lost every ounce of who they are and to get that back is such a struggle.

This is not for you. This is your wake-up call. Are you being true to yourself? Are you living your life in a way that honors your thoughts, feelings, emotions, dreams, and desires? Don't suppress yourself -- express yourself.

CHALLENGE YOURSELF

Look at the environment you're in, the areas of your life, and the people you surround yourself with. Can you fully be yourself in these places, situations, and with these people? Now list the things that are causing you to hold back and dim your light. Why are you doing that?

_____

_____

_____

_____

_____

_____

_____

_____

_____

_____

_____

"Be who you are and say what you feel, because those who mind don't matter, and those who matter don't mind."

Bernard M. Baruch

Chapter 10

Having a Deep Why

What's your reason? Your purpose? What is it that keeps you going, makes you excel, and causes you to push every day? That is your *why*.

I'd like to tell you about my why.

When I was preparing for Kokoro, I trained daily. All this time spent working out was taking time away from my wife and kids, and I started to feel guilty about it. I thought, "Here is my family, supporting me and wanting me to do this, but ultimately I am pulling myself away from them."

This was exactly the opposite of what I wanted and demonstrates the mind shift that I experienced through Warrior.

I challenged myself and asked, "How do I pull my family into my training? How can they be a part of this and do this *with* me?" At the time, my kids were under the age of 10, so I knew that I had to be creative.

My first idea was to bring my son, Jesse Jr., along with me as I ran. He rode his bike beside me as I trained, and it was a way for us to connect. He could see what I was doing while training and it was a way for my son to marry up with what I was doing. He would sometimes bike ahead of me to checkpoints. He'd say, "Come on dad," motivating and inspiring me to do it.

I began to rely on my family for support. If I did a workout they were there with me. My next idea involved evening walks as a family. My wife and kids were all there with me, talking about our day, as I wore a 40lb vest while we walked.

I made my training a family affair. My family was my why, and training with them reminded me that they were my why. I realized at some point I was going to have to leverage this experience to make it through Kokoro. I remember thinking, "I'm not going to quit because my kids are here supporting me, even through training." It was really cool, because they experienced what it felt like to see their dad working hard toward something. And I was able to alleviate guilt, remember my why, and make it a way to bring my family together.

For Kokoro, we had to wear these white t-shirts with our last name screen printed on the front and back. I decided to get one for my son in honor of him training with me. I was proud of him and he was proud to wear it. I remember presenting it to him and said, "You earned this by training with me the last 90 days." It was an incredible moment.

As one of my wife's 90-day challenges, she made a big board for me, featuring these cards with moments spent with my family on it -- it was a visual reminder of my why.

I made it to where it was about them, not just about me completing a physical challenge. My family knew they were my why and we all identified that. I realized that I could do all these things, reach all these goals, and complete 90-day challenges, **but if I didn't incorporate my wife and kids into it, what was the point**?

When the Kokoro challenge got difficult, I brought my thoughts to my wife and kids and got choked up about how they trained with me. I thought about all the walks and runs I did with them right there by my side. It was super powerful to share that experience with my family.

Making it a mission to be a part of each other's lives while on the journey is what it's all about. Connection is everything. By making simple adjustments, I was making my goals part of OUR mission instead of MY mission.

If I gave up during Kokoro, I would feel like I was letting my family down. They knew that they were helping me get ready and they wanted to feel like they were a part of it. I always felt supported in that mission.

One of the big things they talk about in the Warrior program is having a why, identifying it, and then incorporating it. By incorporating my family into my training, it solidified what it meant to have a why. Prior to that, it always felt like it remained surface-level, but not anymore.

How important is a why? It's my opinion that **people who lost their way lost their why.**

When you find your why, you feel joy, happiness and fulfillment. You feel connected to people on a deeper level. Just being able to share with people and being vulnerable is liberating. It's like a wildfire that spreads, and it takes over an entire community of people who then start working together by sharing, collaborating, and supporting.

Right now, I am coaching you, and you're going to take this home and coach your wife and your kids. The goodness spreads. There's a lot more responsibility for me because I'm basically coaching all the people that you're impacting too.

Find your why and center your efforts around it. Trust me, you'll become stronger on every front as a result.

CHALLENGE YOURSELF

What is your why and why does it matter to you? How can you
show those people that matter to you that they are your why?
How can you incorporate your why with your goals?

_____

_____

_____

_____

_____

_____

_____

_____

_____

_____

_____

_____

_____

_____

"Efforts and courage are not enough without purpose and direction."

John F. Kennedy

Chapter 11

Letting Go of Your Identity

What do you cling to in your life? Is it who you are and what you do? Or is it who you *were* and what you *did*? What does it take for a man to let go of what he's known?

I want to share with you my remarkable transformation from drug dealer to trainer, and from trainer to coach.

I was always super competitive growing up and learned about steroids in high school. My dad had testicular cancer and was prescribed steroids for treatment. The first person I ever stole from was him.

I had no idea how to use that first bottle, I just knew that I wanted an athletic edge and other guys at the gym were taking them, so it didn't seem so bad.

While taking steroids, I put on 15-20 pounds in a matter of 6-8 weeks, and my bench press was 315 lbs. I started with one rep and could lift 8 reps of 315 in just a couple of months. I remember getting bigger and that continued on through high school. I excelled in football and sports and all areas of my life.

In college I got into bodybuilding and did my first show at 17 years old. For my age I was a big kid, about 220 at about 11-12% body fat -- there aren't a lot of kids that size.

Before I knew it, I was benching 405 lbs. and squatting over 500 lbs., and I quickly identified as an athlete bodybuilder.

I began selling steroids to kids at school and to guys who I knew wanted them. I was only concerned with making enough money to buy my own. Funny enough, I bought from this guy at the gym who looked like Mr. Clean (he actually used to do the commercials). He was from California and would come up to Spokane every couple of weeks to drop off whatever was needed at the gym and he would head home.

While in college, I stopped temporarily so that I wouldn't get caught and have it interfere with my lifelong goal of playing football.

After college, things got more serious. I started selling again and acquired my supply from a pharmacy in Mexico. I would fly down to Tijuana with cash, the pharmacy would have someone would drive it across the border, and I would fly home with a suitcase full of stuff.

The identity that I adopted next was that of a drug dealer. I added in weed, pain pills, and ecstasy to my inventory. I walked into gyms into the manager's offices with duffle bags, I would set them down, work out, and would come back to find cash in my bags.

Although I had a system, the problem was this -- I was selling steroids to so many people in the gym industry that I couldn't get a job as a trainer. No one would hire me because they all knew me as trouble.

I'll never forget when I was 21, and my parents caught me with $15k in steroids while living at their house. I remember thinking that they weren't that bad because they were constantly being used in bodybuilding circles. I was more fascinated by them than anything, and was more scared of selling weed, ecstasy, and pain pills.

Needless to say, my parents didn't agree, and this was practically the last straw.

It took moving to Seattle in my early 20s to finally settle down. I continued a little bit and then stopped dealing completely once I met my wife, around age 26.

The change started with me and I had to be willing to give up my previous identities of athlete and drug dealer. I began working in a gym as the trainer, not the drug-dealing steroid guy. At first it was hard because I had to figure out how to train and achieve gains without it in my system. It made me a better trainer because I researched the best ways to naturally get results.

So when I got into training, I switched my identity again, and leveraged my past experience to achieve my new goals. I invested in courses, classes, or equipment that no one else had when I opened my own business. I invested in products that were always ahead of the market, like TRX or Bootcamps. I was the first one creating or offering those in our area.

A favorite quote of mine is "Be first or be different, and you will have success. If you can be both, you will be the most successful in your area."

You have to realize who you are and leverage that, but you don't have to still be that same person. It's okay to say, "It's not who I am today." The more you hang onto your old identity, the more people put you in that box. If you remember me from high school and ask, "Are you still that same kid who did steroids?" No dude, I'm not that same guy. People will try to take you back to that place constantly.

Even now as a coach, some people want to see a different identity that *they* remember. They'll say, "I don't like that guy, I want a trainer."

But here's what matters -- *I like who I am now*. Breaking that identity is not only tough mentally, but transition is one of the hardest tasks to overcome.

Through this process I have learned and grown. Nothing was in vain.

The experience ultimately taught me how to hustle. I always would figure out how to find the best source with the best supply. To this day, I will do the same thing around training or coaching, and establish the best contacts and sources in whatever industry I am in.

It also taught me to be a marketer because I had to find guys in the gym who were on steroids, willing to pay, all the while running the risk that this was illegal. It wasn't like selling a car or anything.

Now I'm a Hybrid Entrepreneur, which is like an athlete in the business world.

Yes, I made that up but it's true for me.

I want you to know that your identities -- past, present and future -- are all a part of your story, and that it is never too late to transform into someone new.

CHALLENGE YOURSELF

What is your identity, and does it support the lifestyle that you want to live today? List five qualities that make up your identity. Are they in line with the person you want to become? Or are you the same person you were 10 or 20 years ago? If so, why?

_____

_____

_____

_____

_____

_____

_____

_____

_____

_____

_____

"Knowing yourself is the beginning of all wisdom."

Aristotle

Chapter 12

Believe in Yourself

Have you ever lost belief in yourself? I did. Now, in looking at my life, my gains, my confidence, and my success -- it's hard to believe that I once lost sight of myself and my capabilities.

I owe so much of this sense of believing in myself to my wife, Katie.

I grew up confident, strong, competitive, disciplined and a winner. Once my life went off the rails, I got farther and farther away from who I truly was inside. As a result, I stopped believing in me.

It all started at age 19 when I had my son, then lost my son, was in and out of jail, and underwent domestic violence counseling. This phase of losing myself lasted until I was 25. That's six years of self-belief and self-worth... gone.

Everything turned around one day while working at the gym in Washington state. It was the spring of 2004, I was 25 years old, and was signing two women – sisters -- up for memberships at Pure Fitness. One had beautiful, naturally curly, blonde hair. She particularly caught my eye because she was tall and super attractive, hot even.

I sat the ladies down and said, "With your membership, you get two free training sessions." The one with the curly blond hair said, "Well I want to do them with a hot trainer." I replied, "Well, there are only two trainers here and the other one is on vacation, so you're stuck with me."

The blonde's name was Katie, and we had two very memorable training sessions. Her sister never showed, but I remember Katie doing enough talking for the both of them. She asked me 100 questions, but at the time I couldn't figure out why. I remember thinking, "I'm trying to be professional and she just keeps asking question after question." At the time, I was a bit clueless.

I recall that we were on our second workout and the other trainer walked up. He invited Katie to go golfing, but she didn't really say anything. Once he walked away, she turned to me and asked, "Why don't you ask me out?"

We ended up going on a date that night and the rest is history. Although I was focused on my work and not looking for anyone at the time, when someone believes in you and your life gets better, it's an ultimate sign.

Once I had that realization, I thought, "Oh shit, this is real." And then a couple months later I thought, "Okay I'm going to marry this girl."

From the time I met my wife until the time we got married only a year later, I moved up in the company. I went from trainer to training manager to general manager in one year. From there, I worked at the gym another year and opened up my own business a few years later. Life happens fast.

Katie believed in me more than I believed in myself, and it really empowered me in the next few years. I don't know if I would have believed in myself as much if my wife hadn't believed in me. At the time I wondered, "Why does this girl believe in me so much? What does she see in me?"

She believed in me before I did. Her believing in me made me believe in myself.

Katie's got a lot of energy. She's easy to talk to, be around and easy to get to know. Most people can tell my wife their whole life story in the first 10 minutes of meeting her because that's just her personality.

I think the thing inside of this is that it's one thing to believe in yourself but when other people believe in you too, it's magnified. **Surround yourself with people who believe in you.**

This also goes to show that when you believe in someone, it's important to let them know, encourage, support and cheer them on. Your belief may be the key to uncovering theirs.

When you believe in yourself, nothing is impossible.

CHALLENGE YOURSELF

Who do you believe in? Think of someone who inspires you. What traits does that person have that makes you believe in them? Have you demonstrated that you believe in them? Do you believe in yourself? Why or why not? If you don't believe in yourself as much as you once did, why not? What happened?

_____

_____

_____

_____

_____

_____

_____

_____

_____

_____

"To be a champ you have to believe in yourself when no one else will."

Sugar Ray Robinson

Chapter 13

Listening to the Voice

This book is all about impactful moments in my life that have shaped how I have become the man I've become. With every moment I was provided the opportunity to make a choice. I could stop a habit, start a new path, accept a new truth, or assume a new identity.

The story I'm about to relay to you was one of the more remarkable happenings in my life. It's the story of how at age 39, I met God.

I was recommended to go to training called Impact Training in Salt Lake City, Utah. Although I didn't really know what it was about, this spiritual training opportunity was recommended by Garret White, the man behind Wake Up

Warrior. Garrett advised that I push my fears and assumptions aside and said, *"To get the most out of it, you need to go all in 100% and participate."*

I admit, I immediately went into it thinking that it would be all Mormons, and it was going to be extremely weird. As expected, the first 20 minutes did feel strange. I was scanning the room and felt as if my assumptions were correct about being surrounded by Mormons, some were wearing garments that you could visibly see.

Much to my relief, a guy yelled out "Fuck!" and I realized this wasn't a Mormon event.

Things got going and they asked, "Why are you here?" I immediately stood up and answered, "I'm here because I feel like there's some stuff in my past that I haven't dealt with." They followed with the question, "What is it?" I replied, "I don't know." He instantly said, "That's a lie."

This guy just started going after me. I thought, "Holy shit, what did I sign up for? What's happening?" This guy aggressively coached me and taught, "We say things like 'I don't know' and it stops us from exploring any further. It's a cop out, a dead end."

So we went through this thing for the next 20 mins, and although I broke down, I was still kind of guarded. I definitely didn't want to let this guy in. For the next 6-8 hours I went through this experiential training, unsure of what I would get from it.

We moved on to a feedback session where you simply had to stand in front of someone. They brought me up, of course, because I was dressed well, was athletic, and stuck out like a sore thumb.

He gave me "fake" feedback first, saying that I appeared to be a great guy, with nice clothes, who seemed to have it all together. Then he clarified, "That's not really the feedback we're going to do today. You're guarded, you're protected, you seem all about yourself, you seem cocky, you seem like a punk, and you seem like an asshole."

He unloaded on me for the next few minutes in front of 30-40 people. I remember looking through him, acting like it didn't bother me. He said, "You can continue acting like this doesn't bother you and you won't deal with it." I remember thinking, "Who the fuck are you? You don't know me!"

We broke into groups and did the same activity. My partner said, "I feel ripped off around you." He explained that it was because I was closed off and not sharing.

That night I went back to my hotel room. All of this shit hit me hard and I broke down and cried. I didn't want to be the guy that everyone said I was. It felt wrong and didn't feel like me.

Then I heard the voice of God say, "That's not who you are. It's not who you really are." Confused, I asked, "What does that mean?"

There was no reply.

The next day, I returned to Impact Training. During one of the sessions, I closed my eyes and I saw God enter the room. He tapped me on the shoulder and said, "Jesse I love you." Although I was startled, *it was the first time I felt love for myself*, so it was super powerful.

At the end of the exercise, I got up and shared about the experience. The entire time, I felt God's presence in the room.

Everything kind of started to shift from that place. Although we had to do exercises like beating on chairs to release pain, or jumping up and down singing a song in front of everyone, I carried a new sense of self-love.

I also looked at a guy at the conference and saw he had this bright yellow light shooting out of his neck. After that experience, I could see and read people's energy and their light.

I went from getting my ass kicked emotionally on day one to sharing my positive experience on what I got out of the training at the end of day two. It was a complete 180.

That night I went back to my hotel. I was processing everything that happened over the past couple days and although tired, I was on such a high and I couldn't sleep. I recall being in my bed and I heard a voice say, "Jesse get up and dance with me." Surprised again, I asked, "What is this?" I heard the voice of God again say, "Turn the music on."

For two whole hours, I danced, I talked, and I shared with Him about life. We talked about my life, from moment to moment. It was such a surreal and fulfilling experience.

Knowing that I couldn't keep this to myself, I had to share it with my wife. "You're going to think this is really weird," I said, "but I danced with God last night." Most people wouldn't believe me, but Katie said, "Oh my gosh, that's incredible!"

It was the most powerful experience I've ever had with God and it was the first time I ever felt God come through me. I felt that he was right there and that I could openly communicate and be in line with him.

I kind of always questioned if God was real, but this day removed all doubt. I felt his presence more there than in any church I'd been to.

I think if you don't trust in the man who created you, if you don't believe that there's something more out there, then you don't really trust or believe in yourself.

I think if you believe in something, it gives you a sense of direction and purpose so that you're not just wandering and living life aimlessly. I think there are all kinds of ways to access God. You can sit quietly, talk to Him, meditate, go into the forest, or just be connected with the earth.

I believe that prayer is talking to God, and meditation is listening to God. Look at Him like just another man that you would go to for advice.

I encourage you to find ways to be connected, to dig deeper into your beliefs, and to trust the voice. When you believe in something you'll feel freer, more connected, and you'll realize that you're not alone.

CHALLENGE YOURSELF

Do you believe in yourself? Do you believe in God or a Higher Power? When was the last time you felt connected to God? If you don't believe, think of five things that have happened in your life that you can't explain.

_____

_____

_____

_____

_____

_____

_____

_____

_____

_____

_____

"God gave us the gift of life; it is up to us to give ourselves the gift of living well."

Voltaire

Chapter 14

Modern Money, My Currency

Money. Whether you like it or not, it has a stigma to it. So many of my early opinions on money came from my parents. The negative viewpoint I held for most of my life is incredible, and perhaps you share in some of these beliefs too.

I hope that this chapter will challenge your viewpoints of money and turn them from the negative to the positive. I want to tell you about my breakthrough of discovering that money is love.

I was brought up by parents who were very middle class. My dad would always talk shit about people with money. Having it was fine up to a certain amount. Basically, you could have enough to live off, and maybe a little more to be comfortable, but anything above that was bad. You were selfish, it was the root of all evil -- things I am sure you've heard before. Even when I went to church, I was told that if I didn't tithe, I was bad. Sound familiar?

As I was dealing drugs, I learned about money, but I didn't respect it because it was easy. When I switched to working in gyms, money was hard because I was making almost nothing as a trainer in the beginning. It was so bad that I nearly went broke, and I wasn't sure if I'd be able to continue to do the job.

Once I started having success in the gym world, I educated myself about money and investing. One of the owners of the gyms I worked for brought us to a conference on money and it was eye-opening. One of my favorite takeaways was working towards a goal, saving your money, and allotting it toward a large purpose.

Because of this, I set out to buy a new car. I ended up with a white Chevy Tahoe, it was a 2002 or 2003, and I loved it. It was a super cool car. The day that I finally bought it, I felt so great and so proud.

When I opened my own business, I made more money than ever and built a multi-million-dollar training business. This was nearly unbelievable to me, numbers like these were not seen in my childhood.

While on my path of growth and self-discovery, I decided to completely step out of my comfort zone. Just over nine months ago, I had my energy read by Nancy, a psychic reader. She said that she saw the Eye of Horus and God standing behind me. She told me, "You need to study the Eye of Horus." I didn't know what that was and wondered what the hell she meant.

Coincidentally enough, two days prior, I came across a book called *Money Is Love* by Barbara Wilder and I ordered it.

Now this is where it gets really fascinating.

My book arrived from Amazon, and I opened it randomly to page 55. There it was -- the Eye of Horus. The page was explaining the dollar bill and the meaning of the symbols on it. If you look at a dollar bill right now, on the back you'll see a pyramid and an eye, that's the Eye of Horus. It's an ancient Egyptian symbol of protection, royal power, and good health.

The idea behind *Money is Love* is that money is energy. If you actually trace money back to the earliest of times, it was a different form of currency. It started as grain, then transitioned to silver, and then to gold. The exchange of currency was a spiritual one. Silver represented the moon and gold represented the sun. The simple exchange of grains, plants, food, and coins was how people survived.

The book explains that money is love and love is an energy, and you have to change your energy in order to create more money.

Every time you do business with people, it's simply an exchange of energy. If you do it with the wrong people, it affects your currency.

I began exploring the old beliefs I had about money. That money was bad, evil, and other dark thoughts that were driven from fear and scarcity. I learned from the book that it was only deemed "evil" after it went mainstream.

One of the beliefs that came up in order for me to sell my business, was giving up the belief that my business wasn't worth the money. Once I changed my thinking, it opened me up to selling the business. I was worth it! My business was worth it. Accumulating money didn't mean I was bad, selfish, greedy, or evil. Instead it meant that something I worked hard to build was valued, and someone wanted to exchange energy to make it theirs.

After speaking to Nancy the psychic, and reading the book, my entire way of thinking about money changed.

Money is finite, it's a resource, and we've always had enough money for what we needed. In that essence, I realized that I had a belief that was stopping the flow of money. *It wasn't bad or evil, it was just an exchange of energy.*

Energy is a resource that doesn't go away, it just transfers. Money does the same thing, but we never actually look at it in that aspect. Just think of how different it feels if you hold a $1 dollar bill versus a $100 dollar bill. It's all because of the beliefs we have about money.

Are you ready to change your way of thinking about money? Are you ready to open yourself to the possibility that it is not bad, and that you, your work, your business, and your family are worth it?

CHALLENGE YOURSELF

Sit down in a quiet place with a journal and meditate on your mindset of money for 10 minutes. Now write down all of your stories, beliefs, feelings, and emotions about money. Where did they come from? Are they positive or negative? Are you financially where you thought you'd be at this point? If not, is it because of the negative story you've been telling yourself about money?

"Money is energy that should flow freely through our lives and throughout the world."

Barbara Wilder

Chapter 15

Reflect on Your Reflection

I've taken you on quite a journey and I hope that along the way you have found inspiration and are ready to embrace a new, enriching, challenge-based lifestyle.

If you could picture my reflection through my stories, the corresponding images would vary heavily, yet every reflection is me. The mirror would reveal a cautious boy with an alcoholic father, a determined athlete, a struggling young father in a turbulent relationship, a frustrated man in domestic violence counseling, a drug dealer, a trainer, a committed husband, a hard working entrepreneur, a dedicated father, a coach, and a determined Warrior.

Every single glimpse into the mirror has led to who I am today. Every experience and every lesson brought the opportunity for me to choose a new direction. It's true, some choices led me down paths of destruction, but others led me down paths of discovery.

Just like me, your choices, experiences, relationships and lessons have made you who you are today.

When I think about what brought me through the tough times, the challenges, the races, the seminars, and the life struggles, it was that *I didn't quit.* Sure, there were times I slowed my pace, resorted to escapism, and could have handled things differently. But when I look back to moments of success and victory like pushing myself to my utmost physical and spiritual limits, living a challenge-based lifestyle, and improving in the Core-4 areas of my life, I know I am on the right track.

And now that I have my family, they propel me to push even harder and grow even further. I am immensely grateful for my why.

I want to tell you this -- don't quit. Life gets tough, sometimes we choose the wrong or difficult path, but keep going. Listen to the voice, push yourself, challenge yourself to grow, discover and improve. You're worth it and the lives of those you impact are worth it.

I want you to know that no matter where you are in life or who you identify as, you can refocus and start on a new course at any time. You aren't held to the constraints, thinking, mistakes, labels, or even relationships of your past.

All you have to decide is that you want to live your best life possible and you want to start today. Commit to taking little steps that add up to great ones, and you will find yourself hitting your goals today, tomorrow, and for years to come.

Ask yourself the hard questions, evaluate your life, job, friendships, relationships, and examine what is holding you back. Be honest with yourself and know that you may hit some sore spots and hard moments, but *in your pit is where you find your purpose*.

Once you master challenge-based living, and you set daily intentions for Body, Being, Balance, and Business, you will feel more in control of your life. You will live a purposeful life by choice and by design.

I encourage you to find your inner warrior. Fight for yourself, for your family, and strive to be proud of who you see in the mirror every day.

CHALLENGE YOURSELF

What have you learned through reading this book? What will you implement immediately? What more can you envision for your life? I want you to know that whatever you want is within reach -- you are a warrior.

_____

_____

_____

_____

_____

_____

_____

_____

_____

_____

_____

"The past does not equal the future."

Tony Robbins

To the man in the mirror,

Thank you for reading my book.

If my story has added any value to your life, and if you feel like you're better off after reading it, you have a responsibility.

Please share this message with anyone who needs the guidance or the want to better their life. I hope my story can help you see that the ultimate version of yourself is just on the other side of the challenge in front of you.

If I have done that, then my job is complete.

There is no better way to end this book than with some lyrics from a song that reminds me of the day that my life changed forever. I can still remember my 40th birthday and holding my wife as this song played at the Michael Jackson show in Vegas. I knew things would never be the same. Thankfully, I was right.

We all want change in our life. Only some do something about it.

"I'm starting with the man in the mirror
I'm asking him to change his ways
And no message could have been any clearer
If you want to make the world a better place
Take a look at yourself, and then make a change"

Man in the Mirror

by

Michael Jackson

11505075R00071

Made in the USA
San Bernardino, CA
05 December 2018